ANTI-CANCER DIET COOKBOOK

Nourishing Recipes for a Healthier Tomorrow

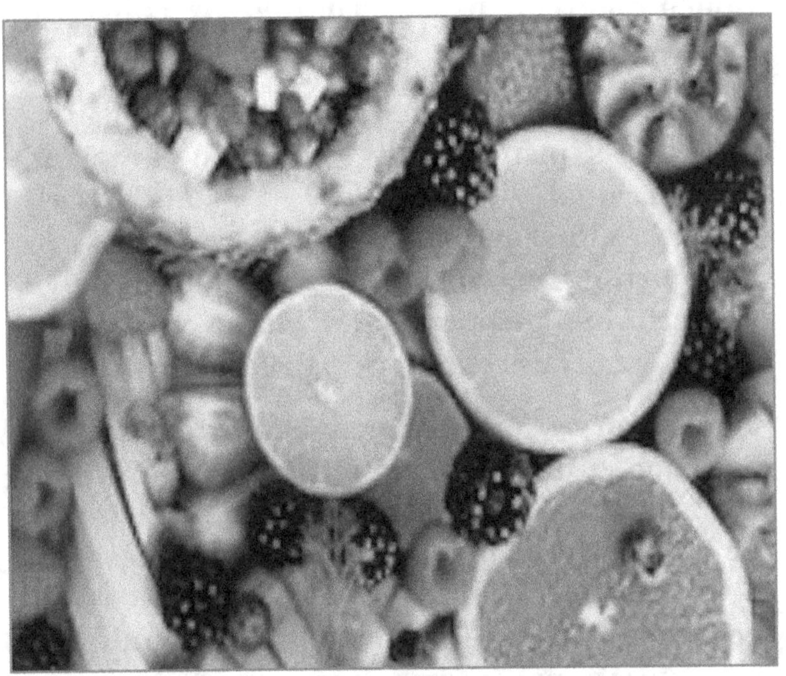

LAUREN WILLS

TABLE OF CONTENT

INTRODUCTION

Welcome to the "Anti-Cancer Diet Cookbook," a collection of wholesome and delicious recipes designed to support your journey towards a healthier and cancer-fighting lifestyle. The power of nutrition in preventing and combatting cancer cannot be overstated, and these recipes have been thoughtfully crafted to provide you with a variety of nutrient-rich, flavorful, and satisfying meals.

Cancer is a formidable adversary, affecting millions of lives worldwide. While medical advancements have made significant strides in cancer treatment, adopting a diet rich in cancer-fighting foods can play a crucial role in reducing the risk of cancer and supporting overall well-being. This cookbook is your culinary companion on this important journey.

Each recipe in this cookbook is more than just a delightful dish; it is a carefully curated selection of ingredients that are known for their cancer-fighting properties. From vibrant vegetables and fruits to lean proteins, whole grains, and beneficial herbs and spices, our recipes encompass a wide range of flavors and textures to keep your meals exciting and nutritious.

Whether you are embarking on a cancer prevention plan, supporting a loved one through their cancer journey, or simply striving for a healthier lifestyle, the "Anti-Cancer Diet Cookbook" is here to empower you with the tools and knowledge to make informed dietary choices.

In addition to delicious recipes, you will find nutritional information for each dish, helping you keep track of your dietary intake. We encourage you to explore the diverse array of recipes within these pages, experiment with new flavors, and, most importantly, prioritize your health.

By incorporating these nutrient-dense recipes into your daily life, you are taking proactive steps to nourish your body and promote overall wellness. Remember, your journey towards a healthier you starts with the choices you make in the kitchen. Here's to your health and well-being!

ANTI-CANCER RECIPES

Recipe 1: Roasted Turmeric Cauliflower

Prep Time: 10 minutes

Serves: 4

Ingredients:

- 1 head cauliflower, cut into florets
- 2 tablespoons olive oil
- 1 teaspoon turmeric powder
- 1/2 teaspoon cumin powder
- Salt and pepper to taste

Directions:

1. Preheat your oven to 425°F (220°C).

2. In a large bowl, combine cauliflower florets, olive oil, turmeric, cumin, salt, and pepper. Toss to coat evenly.

3. Spread the cauliflower in a single layer on a baking sheet.

4. Roast in the oven for 20-25 minutes or until golden brown and tender, stirring halfway through.

5. Serve hot.

Nutritional Value (per serving):

- Calories: 85

- Protein: 3g

- Carbohydrates: 9g

- Fiber: 3g

- Fat: 5g

Recipe 2: Quinoa and Black Bean Salad

Prep Time: 15 minutes

Serves: 4

Ingredients:

- 1 cup quinoa, cooked and cooled

- 1 can (15 oz) black beans, drained and rinsed

- 1 cup cherry tomatoes, halved

- 1/2 cup red onion, finely chopped

- 1/4 cup fresh cilantro, chopped

- 2 tablespoons lime juice

- 2 tablespoons olive oil

- Salt and pepper to taste

Directions:

1. In a large bowl, combine quinoa, black beans, cherry tomatoes, red onion, and cilantro.

2. In a small bowl, whisk together lime juice, olive oil, salt, and pepper.

3. Drizzle the dressing over the salad and toss to combine.

4. Serve chilled.

Nutritional Value (per serving):

- Calories: 270

- Protein: 9g

- Carbohydrates: 42g

- Fiber: 10g

- Fat: 8g

Recipe 3: Baked Salmon with Lemon and Dill

Prep Time: 15 minutes

Serves: 4

Ingredients:

- 4 salmon fillets

- 2 lemons, thinly sliced

- 2 tablespoons fresh dill, chopped

- 2 cloves garlic, minced

- 2 tablespoons olive oil

- Salt and pepper to taste

Directions:

1. Preheat your oven to 375°F (190°C).

2. Place salmon fillets on a baking sheet lined with parchment paper.

3. Season salmon with salt, pepper, and minced garlic.

4. Arrange lemon slices on top of the fillets and sprinkle with fresh dill.

5. Drizzle olive oil over the salmon.

6. Bake for 15-20 minutes or until salmon flakes easily with a fork.

7. Serve with steamed vegetables.

Nutritional Value (per serving):

- Calories: 280

- Protein: 30g

- Carbohydrates: 4g

- Fiber: 1g

- Fat: 16g

Recipe 4: Spinach and Mushroom Stuffed Chicken Breast

Prep Time: 20 minutes

Serves: 4

Ingredients:

- 4 boneless, skinless chicken breasts

- 1 cup spinach, chopped

- 1 cup mushrooms, finely diced

- 1/2 cup low-fat cream cheese

- 2 cloves garlic, minced

- 1 teaspoon olive oil

- Salt and pepper to taste

Directions:

1. Preheat your oven to 375°F (190°C).

2. In a skillet, heat olive oil over medium heat. Add garlic and sauté for 1 minute.

3. Add chopped spinach and mushrooms to the skillet and cook until they release their moisture, about 5 minutes. Season with salt and pepper.

4. Remove the skillet from heat and stir in the cream cheese until well combined.

5. Cut a pocket into each chicken breast and stuff with the spinach and mushroom mixture.

6. Season the outside of the chicken breasts with salt and pepper.

7. Place the stuffed chicken breasts on a baking sheet and bake for 25-30 minutes or until the chicken is cooked through.

8. Serve hot.

Nutritional Value (per serving):

- Calories: 290

- Protein: 38g

- Carbohydrates: 4g

- Fiber: 1g

- Fat: 13g

Recipe 5: Lentil and Vegetable Soup

Prep Time: 30 minutes

Serves: 6

Ingredients:

- 1 cup green or brown lentils, rinsed and drained

- 1 onion, chopped

- 2 carrots, chopped

- 2 celery stalks, chopped

- 2 cloves garlic, minced

- 6 cups vegetable broth

- 1 teaspoon ground cumin

- 1/2 teaspoon paprika

- Salt and pepper to taste

- Fresh parsley for garnish (optional)

Directions:

1. In a large pot, sauté the chopped onion, carrots, celery, and garlic in a bit of olive oil until they start to soften, about 5 minutes.

2. Add lentils, vegetable broth, ground cumin, paprika, salt, and pepper. Bring to a boil.

3. Reduce heat and simmer for 20-25 minutes or until lentils are tender.

4. Serve hot, garnished with fresh parsley if desired.

Nutritional Value (per serving):

- Calories: 180

- Protein: 9g

- Carbohydrates: 33g

- Fiber: 13g

- Fat: 1g

Recipe 6: Grilled Portobello Mushrooms with Balsamic Glaze

Prep Time: 15 minutes

Serves: 4

Ingredients:

- 4 large Portobello mushrooms, stems removed

- 2 tablespoons balsamic vinegar

- 2 tablespoons olive oil

- 2 cloves garlic, minced

- 1 teaspoon dried thyme

- Salt and pepper to taste

- Fresh basil leaves for garnish (optional)

Directions:

1. In a bowl, whisk together balsamic vinegar, olive oil, minced garlic, dried thyme, salt, and pepper.

2. Brush the mixture over both sides of the Portobello mushrooms.

3. Preheat your grill to medium-high heat.

4. Grill the mushrooms for about 4-5 minutes on each side, or until they are tender and grill marks appear.

5. Serve hot, garnished with fresh basil leaves if desired.

Nutritional Value (per serving):

- Calories: 70

- Protein: 3g

- Carbohydrates: 5g

- Fiber: 1g

- Fat: 5g

Recipe 7: Brown Rice and Vegetable Stir-Fry

Prep Time: 20 minutes

Serves: 4

Ingredients:

- 2 cups cooked brown rice

- 1 cup broccoli florets

- 1 cup bell peppers, sliced

- 1 cup snow peas

- 1 carrot, sliced into matchsticks

- 2 cloves garlic, minced

- 2 tablespoons low-sodium soy sauce

- 1 tablespoon sesame oil

- 1 teaspoon grated ginger

- 1/4 cup cashews (optional)

- Sesame seeds for garnish (optional)

Directions:

1. In a large skillet or wok, heat sesame oil over medium-high heat.

2. Add minced garlic and grated ginger, sauté for about 30 seconds.

3. Add broccoli, bell peppers, snow peas, and carrot matchsticks. Stir-fry for 5-7 minutes or until the vegetables are tender.

4. Add cooked brown rice and soy sauce to the skillet. Stir-fry for an additional 2-3 minutes.

5. Serve hot, garnished with cashews and sesame seeds if desired.

Nutritional Value (per serving):

- Calories: 250

- Protein: 7g

- Carbohydrates: 42g

- Fiber: 5g

- Fat: 6g

Recipe 8: Broccoli and Avocado Salad

Prep Time: 15 minutes

Serves: 4

Ingredients:

- 2 cups broccoli florets, blanched

- 2 ripe avocados, diced

- 1/4 cup red onion, finely chopped

- 1/4 cup fresh parsley, chopped

- 2 tablespoons lemon juice

- 2 tablespoons olive oil

- Salt and pepper to taste

- 1/4 cup toasted almond slices for garnish (optional)

Directions:

1. In a large bowl, combine blanched broccoli, diced avocado, chopped red onion, and fresh parsley.

2. In a small bowl, whisk together lemon juice, olive oil, salt, and pepper.

3. Drizzle the dressing over the salad and toss gently to coat.

4. Garnish with toasted almond slices if desired.

5. Serve chilled.

Nutritional Value (per serving):

- Calories: 220

- Protein: 3g

- Carbohydrates: 12g

- Fiber: 7g

- Fat: 19g

Recipe 9: Chickpea and Spinach Curry

Prep Time: 25 minutes

Serves: 4

Ingredients:

- 2 cans (15 oz each) chickpeas, drained and rinsed
- 2 cups fresh spinach
- 1 onion, finely chopped
- 2 cloves garlic, minced
- 1 can (14 oz) diced tomatoes
- 2 tablespoons curry powder
- 1 teaspoon cumin
- 1 teaspoon coriander
- Salt and pepper to taste
- 1 tablespoon olive oil

Directions:

1. In a large skillet, heat olive oil over medium heat. Add chopped onion and minced garlic, sauté until fragrant, about 2 minutes.

2. Stir in curry powder, cumin, and coriander. Cook for an additional 1-2 minutes.

3. Add chickpeas and diced tomatoes (with juice) to the skillet. Simmer for 10 minutes.

4. Stir in fresh spinach and cook until wilted.

5. Season with salt and pepper.

6. Serve hot with brown rice or whole wheat naan.

Nutritional Value (per serving):

- Calories: 290

- Protein: 11g

- Carbohydrates: 49g

- Fiber: 12g

- Fat: 6g

Recipe 10: Grilled Vegetable and Quinoa Stuffed Peppers

Prep Time: 30 minutes

Serves: 4

Ingredients:

- 4 bell peppers, any color

- 1 cup cooked quinoa

- 1 cup grilled vegetables (zucchini, eggplant, bell peppers)

- 1 cup canned black beans, drained and rinsed

- 1/2 cup corn kernels (fresh or frozen)

- 1/2 cup shredded low-fat cheddar cheese (optional)

- 1 teaspoon chili powder

- Salt and pepper to taste

- Olive oil for brushing

Directions:

1. Preheat your grill to medium-high heat.

2. Cut the tops off the bell peppers and remove the seeds and membranes.

3. Brush the outside of the peppers with olive oil and grill for 5-7 minutes per side until slightly charred and tender.

4. In a bowl, combine cooked quinoa, grilled vegetables, black beans, corn, shredded cheese (if using), chili powder, salt, and pepper.

5. Stuff the grilled peppers with the quinoa and vegetable mixture.

6. Place the stuffed peppers back on the grill for 5-7 minutes until the filling is heated through.

7. Serve hot.

Nutritional Value (per serving):

- Calories: 270

- Protein: 10g

- Carbohydrates: 49g

- Fiber: 11g

- Fat: 4g

Recipe 11: Cucumber and Avocado Gazpacho

Prep Time: 15 minutes

Serves: 4

Ingredients:

- 2 cucumbers, peeled and diced

- 2 ripe avocados, peeled and diced

- 1/2 red onion, finely chopped

- 2 cloves garlic, minced

- 3 cups vegetable broth

- 2 tablespoons lime juice

- 2 tablespoons fresh cilantro, chopped

- Salt and pepper to taste

Directions:

1. In a blender, combine diced cucumbers, avocados, chopped red onion, minced garlic, vegetable broth, lime juice, and fresh cilantro.

2. Blend until smooth.

3. Season with salt and pepper.

4. Chill in the refrigerator for at least 30 minutes before serving.

5. Serve cold, garnished with additional cilantro if desired.

Nutritional Value (per serving):

- Calories: 170

- Protein: 3g

- Carbohydrates: 14g

- Fiber: 7g

- Fat: 13g

Recipe 12: Walnut and Kale Pesto Pasta *Prep Time: 20 minutes Serves: 4*

Ingredients:

- 8 oz whole wheat pasta

- 2 cups fresh kale leaves, stems removed

- 1/2 cup walnuts

- 2 cloves garlic, minced

- 1/2 cup grated Parmesan cheese

- 1/4 cup olive oil

- Juice of 1 lemon

- Salt and pepper to taste

Directions:

1. Cook pasta according to package instructions. Drain and set aside.

2. In a food processor, combine kale, walnuts, minced garlic, Parmesan cheese, olive oil, lemon juice, salt, and pepper.

3. Blend until a smooth pesto sauce forms.

4. Toss the cooked pasta with the kale pesto sauce.

5. Serve hot, garnished with additional grated Parmesan if desired.

Nutritional Value (per serving):

- Calories: 480

- Protein: 15g

- Carbohydrates: 38g

- Fiber: 6g

- Fat: 32g

Recipe 13: Spaghetti Squash with Tomato Basil Sauce

Prep Time: 30 minutes

Serves: 4

Ingredients:

- 1 spaghetti squash, halved and seeds removed

- 2 cups tomato sauce (low-sodium)

- 1/4 cup fresh basil leaves, chopped

- 2 cloves garlic, minced

- 1/4 cup grated Parmesan cheese (optional)

- Salt and pepper to taste

Directions:

1. Preheat your oven to 375°F (190°C).

2. Place the halved spaghetti squash on a baking sheet, cut side down.

3. Bake for 25-30 minutes, or until the squash is tender when pierced with a fork.

4. While the squash is baking, in a saucepan, heat the tomato sauce over low heat. Add minced garlic and fresh basil. Simmer for 10 minutes.

5. Use a fork to scrape the cooked spaghetti squash into strands.

6. Serve the squash with the tomato basil sauce and sprinkle with grated Parmesan cheese if desired.

7. Season with salt and pepper.

8. Serve hot.

Nutritional Value (per serving):

- Calories: 90

- Protein: 3g

- Carbohydrates: 16g

- Fiber: 4g

- Fat: 3g

Recipe 14: Berry and Spinach Smoothie

Prep Time: 5 minutes

Serves: 2

Ingredients:

- 2 cups fresh spinach leaves

- 1 cup mixed berries (strawberries, blueberries, raspberries)

- 1 banana

- 1 cup unsweetened almond milk

- 1 tablespoon honey (optional)

Directions:

1. In a blender, combine fresh spinach, mixed berries, banana, and almond milk.

2. Add honey if you prefer a sweeter taste.

3. Blend until smooth.

4. Pour into glasses and serve immediately.

Nutritional Value (per serving):

- Calories: 120

- Protein: 2g

- Carbohydrates: 28g

- Fiber: 5g

- Fat: 1g

Recipe 15: Roasted Beet and Orange Salad

Prep Time: 25 minutes

Serves: 4

Ingredients:

- 4 medium beets, peeled and diced

- 2 oranges, peeled and segmented

- 1/4 cup red onion, thinly sliced

- 1/4 cup fresh mint leaves, chopped

- 2 tablespoons olive oil

- 1 tablespoon balsamic vinegar

- Salt and pepper to taste

Directions:

1. Preheat your oven to 400°F (200°C).

2. Toss diced beets in olive oil and roast for 20-25 minutes, or until tender.

3. In a bowl, combine roasted beets, orange segments, sliced red onion, and chopped mint leaves.

4. Drizzle with balsamic vinegar, season with salt and pepper, and toss gently.

5. Serve chilled.

Nutritional Value (per serving):

- Calories: 120

- Protein: 2g

- Carbohydrates: 19g

- Fiber: 4g

- Fat: 5g

Recipe 16: Tofu and Vegetable Stir-Fry

Prep Time: 20 minutes

Serves: 4

Ingredients:

- 1 block extra-firm tofu, pressed and cubed

- 2 cups broccoli florets

- 1 red bell pepper, sliced

- 1 yellow bell pepper, sliced

- 1 cup snap peas, trimmed

- 2 cloves garlic, minced

- 1/4 cup low-sodium soy sauce

- 2 tablespoons rice vinegar

- 1 tablespoon sesame oil

- 1 tablespoon cornstarch

- 1 tablespoon honey (optional)

- Sesame seeds for garnish (optional)

Directions:

1. In a bowl, whisk together soy sauce, rice vinegar, sesame oil, cornstarch, and honey (if using). Set aside.

2. In a large skillet or wok, heat a bit of olive oil over medium-high heat.

3. Add cubed tofu and stir-fry until golden brown, about 5-7 minutes. Remove tofu from the skillet and set aside.

4. In the same skillet, add a bit more olive oil if needed and sauté minced garlic for 30 seconds.

5. Add broccoli, red bell pepper, yellow bell pepper, and snap peas. Stir-fry for 5-7 minutes or until vegetables are tender.

6. Return the tofu to the skillet and pour the sauce over the tofu and vegetables.

7. Stir-fry for an additional 2-3 minutes until the sauce thickens.

8. Garnish with sesame seeds if desired.

9. Serve hot over brown rice or quinoa.

Nutritional Value (per serving):

- Calories: 240

- Protein: 15g

- Carbohydrates: 24g

- Fiber: 4g

- Fat: 11g

Recipe 17: Lemon Garlic Shrimp with Asparagus

Prep Time: 15 minutes

Serves: 4

Ingredients:

- 1 pound large shrimp, peeled and deveined

- 1 bunch asparagus, trimmed and cut into 2-inch pieces

- 3 cloves garlic, minced

- 2 tablespoons olive oil

- Juice and zest of 1 lemon

- 1 teaspoon dried oregano

- Salt and pepper to taste

- Fresh parsley for garnish (optional)

Directions:

1. In a bowl, combine shrimp, minced garlic, olive oil, lemon juice, lemon zest, dried oregano, salt, and pepper. Toss to coat.

2. Heat a large skillet over medium-high heat.

3. Add the shrimp and cook for 1-2 minutes per side until pink and cooked through. Remove from the skillet and set aside.

4. In the same skillet, add a bit more olive oil if needed and sauté asparagus for 4-5 minutes until tender.

5. Return the cooked shrimp to the skillet and toss with the asparagus.

6. Garnish with fresh parsley if desired.

7. Serve hot.

Nutritional Value (per serving):

- Calories: 190

- Protein: 22g

- Carbohydrates: 5g

- Fiber: 2g

- Fat: 9g

Recipe 18: Sweet Potato and Black Bean Tacos

Prep Time: 30 minutes

Serves: 4

Ingredients:

- 2 medium sweet potatoes, peeled and diced

- 1 can (15 oz) black beans, drained and rinsed

- 1 teaspoon chili powder

- 1/2 teaspoon cumin

- 1/2 teaspoon paprika

- Salt and pepper to taste

- 8 small whole wheat tortillas

- Salsa, avocado, and cilantro for toppings

Directions:

1. Preheat your oven to 425°F (220°C).

2. Toss sweet potato cubes with olive oil, chili powder, cumin, paprika, salt, and pepper. Spread on a baking sheet and roast for 20-25 minutes until tender.

3. In a small saucepan, heat black beans over medium-low heat. Season with a pinch of salt and pepper.

4. Warm tortillas in a dry skillet or microwave.

5. Assemble tacos by filling each tortilla with roasted sweet potatoes, black beans, salsa, avocado, and cilantro.

6. Serve warm.

Nutritional Value (per serving):

- Calories: 320

- Protein: 9g

- Carbohydrates: 60g

- Fiber: 11g

- Fat: 5g

Recipe 19: Mediterranean Chickpea Salad

Prep Time: 20 minutes

Serves: 4

Ingredients:

- 2 cans (15 oz each) chickpeas, drained and rinsed

- 1 cucumber, diced

- 1 cup cherry tomatoes, halved

- 1/2 cup red onion, finely chopped

- 1/4 cup fresh parsley, chopped

- 1/4 cup Kalamata olives, pitted and sliced

- 1/4 cup feta cheese, crumbled (optional)

- Juice of 1 lemon

- 2 tablespoons extra-virgin olive oil

- 1 teaspoon dried oregano

- Salt and pepper to taste

Directions:

1. In a large bowl, combine chickpeas, diced cucumber, halved cherry tomatoes, chopped red onion, chopped parsley, sliced Kalamata olives, and crumbled feta cheese (if using).

2. In a small bowl, whisk together lemon juice, extra-virgin olive oil, dried oregano, salt, and pepper.

3. Drizzle the dressing over the salad and toss gently to combine.

4. Serve chilled.

Nutritional Value (per serving):

- Calories: 280

- Protein: 11g

- Carbohydrates: 37g

- Fiber: 11g

- Fat: 11g

Recipe 20: Stuffed Bell Peppers with Quinoa and Black Beans

Prep Time: 30 minutes

Serves: 4

Ingredients:

- 4 bell peppers, any color

- 1 cup cooked quinoa

- 1 can (15 oz) black beans, drained and rinsed

- 1 cup corn kernels (fresh or frozen)

- 1 cup diced tomatoes

- 1/2 cup diced red onion

- 1 teaspoon chili powder

- 1/2 teaspoon cumin

- Salt and pepper to taste

- 1/2 cup shredded low-fat cheddar cheese (optional)

Directions:

1. Preheat your oven to 375°F (190°C).

2. Cut the tops off the bell peppers and remove the seeds and membranes.

3. In a large bowl, combine cooked quinoa, black beans, corn, diced tomatoes, diced red onion, chili powder, cumin, salt, and pepper.

4. Stuff the bell peppers with the quinoa and black bean mixture.

5. Place the stuffed peppers in a baking dish and cover with aluminum foil.

6. Bake for 25-30 minutes, or until the peppers are tender.

7. Remove the foil and sprinkle shredded cheese (if using) on top of each pepper.

8. Bake for an additional 5-7 minutes, or until the cheese is melted and bubbly.

9. Serve hot.

Nutritional Value (per serving):

- Calories: 290

- Protein: 13g

- Carbohydrates: 55g

- Fiber: 13g

- Fat: 4g

Recipe 21: Berry and Chia Seed Pudding

Prep Time: 10 minutes (plus chilling time)

Serves: 4

Ingredients:

- 1 cup mixed berries (strawberries, blueberries, raspberries)

- 1 cup almond milk (unsweetened)

- 1/4 cup chia seeds

- 2 tablespoons honey (optional)

- 1 teaspoon vanilla extract

Directions:

1. In a blender, combine mixed berries, almond milk, honey (if using), and vanilla extract. Blend until smooth.

2. In a bowl, stir in chia seeds into the berry mixture.

3. Cover and refrigerate for at least 4 hours or overnight until the chia seeds have absorbed the liquid and the mixture has thickened.

4. Serve chilled, garnished with additional berries if desired.

Nutritional Value (per serving):

- Calories: 150

- Protein: 4g

- Carbohydrates: 18g

- Fiber: 8g

- Fat: 7g

Recipe 22: Garlic and Herb Baked Cod

Prep Time: 20 minutes

Serves: 4

Ingredients:

- 4 cod fillets

- 2 tablespoons olive oil

- 4 cloves garlic, minced

- 1 tablespoon fresh thyme leaves

- 1 tablespoon fresh rosemary, chopped

- Zest and juice of 1 lemon

- Salt and pepper to taste

Directions:

1. Preheat your oven to 375°F (190°C).

2. Place the cod fillets in a baking dish.

3. In a small bowl, mix together olive oil, minced garlic, fresh thyme, chopped rosemary, lemon zest, lemon juice, salt, and pepper.

4. Pour the herb mixture over the cod fillets.

5. Bake in the preheated oven for 15-20 minutes or until the fish flakes easily with a fork.

6. Serve hot with steamed vegetables.

Nutritional Value (per serving):

- Calories: 190

- Protein: 26g

- Carbohydrates: 2g

- Fiber: 1g

- Fat: 8g

Recipe 23: Greek Salad with Quinoa

Prep Time: 20 minutes

Serves: 4

Ingredients:

- 2 cups cooked quinoa, cooled

- 1 cucumber, diced

- 1 cup cherry tomatoes, halved

- 1/2 cup Kalamata olives, pitted and sliced

- 1/4 cup red onion, finely chopped

- 1/4 cup crumbled feta cheese

- 1/4 cup fresh parsley, chopped

- 2 tablespoons extra-virgin olive oil

- Juice of 1 lemon

- Salt and pepper to taste

Directions:

1. In a large bowl, combine cooked quinoa, diced cucumber, halved cherry tomatoes, sliced Kalamata olives, chopped red onion, crumbled feta cheese, and chopped fresh parsley.

2. In a small bowl, whisk together extra-virgin olive oil, lemon juice, salt, and pepper.

3. Drizzle the dressing over the salad and toss gently to combine.

4. Serve chilled.

Nutritional Value (per serving):

- Calories: 270

- Protein: 8g

- Carbohydrates: 31g

- Fiber: 5g

- Fat: 14g

Recipe 24: Roasted Butternut Squash Soup

Prep Time: 30 minute

Serves: 6

Ingredients:

- 1 butternut squash, peeled and diced

- 1 onion, chopped

- 2 carrots, chopped

- 2 cloves garlic, minced

- 4 cups vegetable broth

- 1 teaspoon ground cinnamon

- 1/2 teaspoon ground nutmeg

- Salt and pepper to taste

- Greek yogurt for garnish (optional)

Directions:

1. Preheat your oven to 400°F (200°C).

2. Place diced butternut squash, chopped onion, chopped carrots, and minced garlic on a baking sheet.

3. Drizzle with olive oil, sprinkle with ground cinnamon, ground nutmeg, salt, and pepper.

4. Roast in the oven for 25-30 minutes or until vegetables are tender and slightly caramelized.

5. Transfer the roasted vegetables to a large pot, add vegetable broth, and bring to a simmer.

6. Use an immersion blender to puree the soup until smooth. Alternatively, blend in batches in a regular blender.

7. Season with additional salt and pepper if needed.

8. Serve hot, garnished with a dollop of Greek yogurt if desired.

Nutritional Value (per serving):

- Calories: 110

- Protein: 2g

- Carbohydrates: 28g

- Fiber: 5g

- Fat: 1g

Recipe 25: Blueberry and Almond Oatmeal

Prep Time: 10 minutes

Serves: 4

Ingredients:

- 2 cups rolled oats

- 4 cups almond milk (unsweetened)

- 1 cup fresh blueberries

- 1/4 cup sliced almonds

- 2 tablespoons honey (optional)

- 1 teaspoon vanilla extract

- Pinch of salt

Directions:

1. In a saucepan, combine rolled oats, almond milk, honey (if using), vanilla extract, and a pinch of salt.

2. Cook over medium heat, stirring occasionally, until the oatmeal reaches your desired consistency (about 5-7 minutes).

3. Remove from heat and stir in fresh blueberries.

4. Serve hot, garnished with sliced almonds.

Nutritional Value (per serving):

- Calories: 240

- Protein: 6g

- Carbohydrates: 39g

- Fiber: 6g

- Fat: 7g

Recipe 26: Garlic and Ginger Broccoli

Prep Time: 15 minutes

Serves: 4

Ingredients:

- 1 pound broccoli florets

- 2 tablespoons olive oil

- 3 cloves garlic, minced

- 1 tablespoon fresh ginger, grated

- 2 tablespoons low-sodium soy sauce

- 1 teaspoon sesame seeds (optional)

Directions:

1. Steam or blanch the broccoli until tender, about 4-5 minutes. Drain and set aside.

2. In a large skillet, heat olive oil over medium heat. Add minced garlic and grated ginger, sauté for 1-2 minutes.

3. Add the steamed broccoli and soy sauce to the skillet. Toss to coat.

4. Sauté for an additional 2-3 minutes.

5. Sprinkle with sesame seeds if desired.

6. Serve hot.

Nutritional Value (per serving):

- Calories: 80

- Protein: 3g

- Carbohydrates: 8g

- Fiber: 3g

- Fat: 5g

Recipe 27: Grilled Eggplant and Red Pepper Salad

Prep Time: 20 minutes

Serves: 4

Ingredients:

- 2 medium eggplants, sliced

- 2 red bell peppers, halved and seeded

- 1/4 cup fresh basil leaves, chopped

- 2 cloves garlic, minced

- 2 tablespoons balsamic vinegar

- 2 tablespoons extra-virgin olive oil

- Salt and pepper to taste

Directions:

1. Preheat your grill to medium-high heat.

2. Brush eggplant slices and red pepper halves with olive oil.

3. Grill eggplant for 3-4 minutes per side and red peppers for 4-5 minutes per side, until tender and slightly charred.

4. Remove from the grill and let cool slightly.

5. Slice grilled eggplant into strips and chop the grilled red peppers.

6. In a bowl, combine eggplant, red peppers, chopped basil, minced garlic, balsamic vinegar, extra-virgin olive oil, salt, and pepper.

7. Toss gently to combine.

8. Serve chilled or at room temperature.

Nutritional Value (per serving):

- Calories: 100

- Protein: 2g

- Carbohydrates: 13g

- Fiber: 6g

- Fat: 6g

Recipe 28: Almond-Crusted Salmon

Prep Time: 20 minutes

Serves: 4

Ingredients:

- 4 salmon fillets

- 1/2 cup almonds, finely chopped

- 2 tablespoons Dijon mustard

- 1 tablespoon honey

- 1 teaspoon lemon zest

- Salt and pepper to taste

- Lemon wedges for garnish

Directions:

1. Preheat your oven to 375°F (190°C).

2. In a bowl, mix chopped almonds, Dijon mustard, honey, lemon zest, salt, and pepper.

3. Place salmon fillets on a baking sheet lined with parchment paper.

4. Spread the almond mixture evenly over the top of each salmon fillet.

5. Bake for 15-20 minutes or until the salmon flakes easily with a fork.

6. Garnish with lemon wedges and serve hot.

Nutritional Value (per serving):

- Calories: 300

- Protein: 25g

- Carbohydrates: 8g

- Fiber: 2g

- Fat: 20g

Recipe 29: Spinach and Strawberry Salad with Poppy Seed Dressing

Prep Time: 15 minutes

Serves: 4

Ingredients:

- 6 cups baby spinach leaves

- 1 cup strawberries, sliced

- 1/4 cup red onion, thinly sliced

- 1/4 cup slivered almonds, toasted

- 1/4 cup feta cheese, crumbled (optional)

- 2 tablespoons poppy seed dressing

Directions:

1. In a large bowl, combine baby spinach, sliced strawberries, thinly sliced red onion, and toasted slivered almonds.

2. If desired, sprinkle with crumbled feta cheese.

3. Drizzle with poppy seed dressing and toss gently to coat.

4. Serve chilled.

Nutritional Value (per serving):

- Calories: 140

- Protein: 4g

- Carbohydrates: 12g

- Fiber: 3g

- Fat: 9g

Recipe 30: Carrot and Ginger Soup

Prep Time: 30 minutes

Serves: 6

Ingredients:

- 6 large carrots, peeled and chopped

- 1 onion, chopped

- 2 cloves garlic, minced

- 2 tablespoons fresh ginger, grated

- 4 cups vegetable broth

- 1 can (14 oz) coconut milk (unsweetened)

- 1 tablespoon olive oil

- Salt and pepper to taste

- Fresh cilantro for garnish (optional)

Directions:

1. In a large pot, heat olive oil over medium heat. Add chopped onion and minced garlic, sauté for 2-3 minutes.

2. Add chopped carrots and grated ginger to the pot. Sauté for an additional 5 minutes.

3. Pour in vegetable broth and bring to a simmer. Cook until carrots are tender, about 15 minutes.

4. Use an immersion blender to puree the soup until smooth. Alternatively, blend in batches in a regular blender.

5. Return the soup to the pot, add coconut milk, and heat gently.

6. Season with salt and pepper.

7. Garnish with fresh cilantro if desired.

8. Serve hot.

Nutritional Value (per serving):

- Calories: 190

- Protein: 2g

- Carbohydrates: 13g

- Fiber: 4g

- Fat: 14g

Recipe 31: Quinoa and Black Bean Stuffed Peppers

Prep Time: 30 minutes

Serves: 4

Ingredients:

- 4 bell peppers, any color

- 1 cup cooked quinoa

- 1 can (15 oz) black beans, drained and rinsed

- 1 cup corn kernels (fresh or frozen)

- 1 cup diced tomatoes

- 1/2 cup diced red onion

- 1 teaspoon chili powder

- 1/2 teaspoon cumin

- Salt and pepper to taste

- 1/2 cup shredded low-fat cheddar cheese (optional)

Directions:

1. Preheat your oven to 375°F (190°C).

2. Cut the tops off the bell peppers and remove the seeds and membranes.

3. In a large bowl, combine cooked quinoa, black beans, corn, diced tomatoes, diced red onion, chili powder, cumin, salt, and pepper.

4. Stuff the bell peppers with the quinoa and black bean mixture.

5. Place the stuffed peppers in a baking dish and cover with aluminum foil.

6. Bake for 25-30 minutes, or until the peppers are tender.

7. Remove the foil and sprinkle shredded cheese (if using) on top of each pepper.

8. Bake for an additional 5-7 minutes, or until the cheese is melted and bubbly.

9. Serve hot.

Nutritional Value (per serving):

- Calories: 290

- Protein: 13g

- Carbohydrates: 55g

- Fiber: 13g

- Fat: 4g

Recipe 32: Asian-Inspired Tofu Stir-Fry

Prep Time: 25 minutes

Serves: 4

Ingredients:

- 1 block extra-firm tofu, pressed and cubed

- 2 cups broccoli florets

- 1 red bell pepper, sliced

- 1 yellow bell pepper, sliced

- 1 cup snap peas, trimmed

- 2 cloves garlic, minced

- 1/4 cup low-sodium soy sauce

- 2 tablespoons hoisin sauce

- 1 tablespoon rice vinegar

- 1 tablespoon sesame oil

- 1 tablespoon cornstarch

- 1 tablespoon honey (optional)

- Sesame seeds for garnish (optional)

Directions:

1. In a bowl, whisk together soy sauce, hoisin sauce, rice vinegar, sesame oil, cornstarch, and honey (if using). Set aside.

2. In a large skillet or wok, heat a bit of olive oil over medium-high heat.

3. Add cubed tofu and stir-fry until golden brown, about 5-7 minutes. Remove tofu from the skillet and set aside.

4. In the same skillet, add a bit more olive oil if needed and sauté minced garlic for 30 seconds.

5. Add broccoli, red bell pepper, yellow bell pepper, and snap peas. Stir-fry for 5-7 minutes or until vegetables are tender.

6. Return the tofu to the skillet and pour the sauce over the tofu and vegetables.

7. Stir-fry for an additional 2-3 minutes until the sauce thickens.

8. Garnish with sesame seeds if desired.

9. Serve hot over brown rice or quinoa.

Nutritional Value (per serving):

- Calories: 240

- Protein: 15g

- Carbohydrates: 24g

- Fiber: 4g

- Fat: 11g

Recipe 33: Lemon Garlic Shrimp with Zucchini Noodles

Prep Time: 20 minutes

Serves: 4

Ingredients:

- 1 pound large shrimp, peeled and deveined

- 4 medium zucchinis, spiralized into noodles

- 3 cloves garlic, minced

- 2 tablespoons olive oil

- Juice and zest of 1 lemon

- 1 teaspoon dried oregano

- Salt and pepper to taste

- Fresh parsley for garnish (optional)

Directions:

1. In a bowl, combine shrimp, minced garlic, olive oil, lemon juice, lemon zest, dried oregano, salt, and pepper. Toss to coat.

2. Heat a large skillet over medium-high heat.

3. Add the shrimp and cook for 1-2 minutes per side until pink and cooked through. Remove from the skillet and set aside.

4. In the same skillet, add a bit more olive oil if needed and sauté zucchini noodles for 2-3 minutes until tender.

5. Return the cooked shrimp to the skillet and toss with the zucchini noodles.

6. Garnish with fresh parsley if desired.

7. Serve hot.

Nutritional Value (per serving):

- Calories: 180

- Protein: 23g

- Carbohydrates: 8g

- Fiber: 2g

- Fat: 8g

Recipe 34: Roasted Brussels Sprouts with Cranberries and Pecans

Prep Time: 25 minutes

Serves: 4

Ingredients:

- 1 pound Brussels sprouts, trimmed and halved

- 1/2 cup dried cranberries

- 1/2 cup pecans, chopped

- 2 tablespoons olive oil

- 2 tablespoons balsamic vinegar

- 1 tablespoon honey

- Salt and pepper to taste

Directions:

1. Preheat your oven to 400°F (200°C).

2. In a large bowl, toss Brussels sprouts with olive oil, salt, and pepper.

3. Spread the Brussels sprouts on a baking sheet and roast for 20-25 minutes, or until tender and slightly crispy.

4. In a small bowl, mix balsamic vinegar and honey.

5. In a serving bowl, combine roasted Brussels sprouts, dried cranberries, and chopped pecans.

6. Drizzle the balsamic vinegar and honey mixture over the top and toss gently to coat.

7. Serve warm.

Nutritional Value (per serving):

- Calories: 260

- Protein: 4g

- Carbohydrates: 32g

- Fiber: 6g

- Fat: 14g

Recipe 35: Quinoa and Black Bean Stuffed Sweet Potatoes

Prep Time: 45 minutes

Serves: 4

Ingredients:

- 4 medium sweet potatoes

- 1 cup cooked quinoa

- 1 can (15 oz) black beans, drained and rinsed

- 1 cup corn kernels (fresh or frozen)

- 1 cup diced tomatoes

- 1/2 cup diced red onion

- 1 teaspoon chili powder

- 1/2 teaspoon cumin

- Salt and pepper to taste

- 1/2 cup Greek yogurt for topping (optional)

Directions:

1. Preheat your oven to 400°F (200°C).

2. Prick sweet potatoes with a fork and place them on a baking sheet.

3. Bake for 40-45 minutes, or until sweet potatoes are tender.

4. While the sweet potatoes are baking, in a large bowl, combine cooked quinoa, black beans, corn, diced tomatoes, diced red onion, chili powder, cumin, salt, and pepper.

5. Slice each sweet potato open and fluff the flesh with a fork.

6. Stuff the sweet potatoes with the quinoa and black bean mixture.

7. Top with a dollop of Greek yogurt if desired.

8. Serve hot.

Nutritional Value (per serving):

- Calories: 270

- Protein: 11g

- Carbohydrates: 52g

- Fiber: 11g

- Fat: 2g

Recipe 36: Mixed Berry Quinoa Breakfast Bowl

Prep Time: 10 minutes

Serves: 2

Ingredients:

- 1 cup cooked quinoa, cooled

- 1 cup mixed berries (strawberries, blueberries, raspberries)

- 1/4 cup Greek yogurt (unsweetened)

- 2 tablespoons honey

- 2 tablespoons chopped nuts (almonds, walnuts, or pecans)

- 1 teaspoon chia seeds (optional)

Directions:

1. In a bowl, divide cooked quinoa evenly between two servings.

2. Top each bowl with mixed berries, Greek yogurt, honey, chopped nuts, and chia seeds (if using).

3. Serve chilled.

Nutritional Value (per serving):

- Calories: 280

- Protein: 9g

- Carbohydrates: 53g

- Fiber: 7g

- Fat: 6g

Recipe 37: Lentil and Vegetable Soup

Prep Time: 30 minutes

Serves: 6

Ingredients:

- 1 cup green or brown lentils, rinsed and drained

- 1 onion, chopped

- 2 carrots, chopped

- 2 celery stalks, chopped

- 2 cloves garlic, minced

- 4 cups vegetable broth

- 1 can (14 oz) diced tomatoes

- 1 teaspoon dried thyme

- 1 teaspoon dried rosemary

- Salt and pepper to taste

- Fresh parsley for garnish (optional)

Directions:

1. In a large pot, sauté chopped onion, chopped carrots, chopped celery, and minced garlic in a bit of olive oil until vegetables begin to soften, about 5 minutes.

2. Add rinsed lentils, vegetable broth, diced tomatoes, dried thyme, dried rosemary, salt, and pepper to the pot.

3. Bring to a boil, then reduce heat and simmer for 20-25 minutes, or until lentils are tender.

4. Serve hot, garnished with fresh parsley if desired.

Nutritional Value (per serving):

- Calories: 230

- Protein: 13g

- Carbohydrates: 43g

- Fiber: 14g

- Fat: 1g

Recipe 38: Baked Sweet Potato Fries

Prep Time: 25 minutes

Serves: 4

Ingredients:

- 4 medium sweet potatoes, peeled and cut into fries

- 2 tablespoons olive oil

- 1 teaspoon smoked paprika

- 1/2 teaspoon garlic powder

- Salt and pepper to taste

- Greek yogurt or hummus for dipping (optional)

Directions:

1. Preheat your oven to 425°F (220°C).

2. In a large bowl, toss sweet potato fries with olive oil, smoked paprika, garlic powder, salt, and pepper.

3. Spread the fries in a single layer on a baking sheet.

4. Bake for 20-25 minutes, flipping once halfway through, until fries are crispy and golden brown.

5. Serve hot with Greek yogurt or hummus for dipping if desired.

Nutritional Value (per serving):

- Calories: 180

- Protein: 2g

- Carbohydrates: 30g

- Fiber: 5g

- Fat: 7g

Recipe 39: Quinoa and Vegetable Stir-Fry

Prep Time: 25 minutes

Serves: 4

Ingredients:

- 1 cup cooked quinoa

- 2 cups mixed vegetables (broccoli, bell peppers, snap peas)

- 1 cup tofu, cubed

- 2 cloves garlic, minced

- 2 tablespoons low-sodium soy sauce

- 1 tablespoon sesame oil

- 1 tablespoon rice vinegar

- 1 teaspoon honey (optional)

- Sesame seeds for garnish (optional)

Directions:

1. In a bowl, whisk together soy sauce, sesame oil, rice vinegar, and honey (if using). Set aside.

2. In a large skillet or wok, heat a bit of olive oil over medium-high heat.

3. Add cubed tofu and stir-fry until golden brown, about 5-7 minutes. Remove tofu from the skillet and set aside.

4. In the same skillet, add a bit more olive oil if needed and sauté minced garlic for 30 seconds.

5. Add mixed vegetables and stir-fry for 5-7 minutes until tender.

6. Return the tofu to the skillet and pour the sauce over the tofu and vegetables.

7. Stir-fry for an additional 2-3 minutes until the sauce thickens.

8. Garnish with sesame seeds if desired.

9. Serve hot over cooked quinoa.

Nutritional Value (per serving):

- Calories: 260

- Protein: 13g

- Carbohydrates: 30g

- Fiber: 5g

- Fat: 10g

Recipe 40: Baked Cod with Tomato and Olive Relish

Prep Time: 25 minutes

Serves: 4

Ingredients:

- 4 cod fillets

- 1 cup cherry tomatoes, halved

- 1/2 cup Kalamata olives, pitted and sliced

- 2 cloves garlic, minced

- 2 tablespoons extra-virgin olive oil

- 1 tablespoon balsamic vinegar

- 1 teaspoon dried oregano

- Salt and pepper to taste

- Fresh basil for garnish (optional)

Directions:

1. Preheat your oven to 375°F (190°C).

2. In a bowl, combine cherry tomatoes, sliced Kalamata olives, minced garlic, extra-virgin olive oil, balsamic vinegar, dried oregano, salt, and pepper.

3. Place cod fillets on a baking sheet lined with parchment paper.

4. Spoon the tomato and olive relish mixture over the top of each cod fillet.

5. Bake for 15-20 minutes, or until the fish flakes easily with a fork.

6. Garnish with fresh basil if desired.

7. Serve hot.

Nutritional Value (per serving):

- Calories: 220

- Protein: 27g

- Carbohydrates: 5g

- Fiber: 1g

- Fat: 10g

Recipe 41: Quinoa and Kale Salad with Lemon Tahini Dressing

Prep Time: 20 minutes

Serves: 4

Ingredients:

- 2 cups cooked quinoa, cooled

- 4 cups kale leaves, stemmed and chopped

- 1 cup cherry tomatoes, halved

- 1/4 cup red onion, thinly sliced

- 1/4 cup roasted chickpeas (store-bought or homemade)

- 1/4 cup feta cheese, crumbled (optional)

- Juice of 1 lemon

- 2 tablespoons tahini

- 1 clove garlic, minced

- Salt and pepper to taste

Directions:

1. In a large bowl, combine cooked quinoa, chopped kale, halved cherry tomatoes, thinly sliced red onion, roasted chickpeas, and crumbled feta cheese (if using).

2. In a small bowl, whisk together lemon juice, tahini, minced garlic, salt, and pepper.

3. Drizzle the lemon tahini dressing over the salad and toss gently to combine.

4. Serve chilled.

Nutritional Value (per serving):

- Calories: 270

- Protein: 10g

- Carbohydrates: 35g

- Fiber: 5g

- Fat: 10g

Recipe 42: Avocado and Black Bean Salad

Prep Time: 15 minutes

Serves: 4

Ingredients:

- 2 avocados, diced

- 1 can (15 oz) black beans, drained and rinsed

- 1 cup corn kernels (fresh or frozen)

- 1/2 cup red onion, finely chopped

- 1/4 cup fresh cilantro, chopped

- Juice of 2 limes

- 2 tablespoons extra-virgin olive oil

- Salt and pepper to taste

Directions:

1. In a large bowl, combine diced avocados, drained black beans, corn kernels, chopped red onion, and chopped cilantro.

2. In a small bowl, whisk together lime juice, extra-virgin olive oil, salt, and pepper.

3. Drizzle the dressing over the salad and toss gently to combine.

4. Serve chilled.

Nutritional Value (per serving):

- Calories: 290

- Protein: 7g

- Carbohydrates: 29g

- Fiber: 11g

- Fat: 18g

Recipe 43: Lemon Garlic Roasted Chicken

Prep Time: 15 minutes

Serves: 4

Ingredients:

- 4 boneless, skinless chicken breasts

- 4 cloves garlic, minced

- Juice and zest of 2 lemons

- 2 tablespoons olive oil

- 1 teaspoon dried oregano

- Salt and pepper to taste

- Fresh parsley for garnish (optional)

Directions:

1. Preheat your oven to 375°F (190°C).

2. In a bowl, combine minced garlic, lemon juice, lemon zest, olive oil, dried oregano, salt, and pepper.

3. Place chicken breasts in a baking dish.

4. Pour the lemon garlic mixture over the chicken.

5. Bake in the preheated oven for 25-30 minutes, or until the chicken is cooked through.

6. Garnish with fresh parsley if desired.

7. Serve hot.

Nutritional Value (per serving):

- Calories: 220

- Protein: 27g

- Carbohydrates: 2g

- Fiber: 0g

- Fat: 10g

Recipe 44: Quinoa and Mango Salad

Prep Time: 20 minutes

Serves: 4

Ingredients:

- 2 cups cooked quinoa, cooled

- 1 large mango, diced

- 1 red bell pepper, diced

- 1/4 cup red onion, finely chopped

- 1/4 cup fresh cilantro, chopped

- Juice of 2 limes

- 2 tablespoons extra-virgin olive oil

- Salt and pepper to taste

Directions:

1. In a large bowl, combine cooked quinoa, diced mango, diced red bell pepper, finely chopped red onion, and chopped cilantro.

2. In a small bowl, whisk together lime juice, extra-virgin olive oil, salt, and pepper.

3. Drizzle the dressing over the salad and toss gently to combine.

4. Serve chilled.

Nutritional Value (per serving):

- Calories: 280

- Protein: 5g

- Carbohydrates: 46g

- Fiber: 5g

- Fat: 9g

Recipe 45: Chickpea and Vegetable Curry

Prep Time: 30 minutes

Serves: 4

Ingredients:

- 2 cups cooked chickpeas (canned or cooked from dried)

- 2 cups mixed vegetables (bell peppers, zucchini, cauliflower)

- 1 onion, chopped

- 2 cloves garlic, minced

- 1 can (14 oz) diced tomatoes

- 1 can (14 oz) coconut milk (unsweetened)

- 2 tablespoons curry powder

- 1 teaspoon cumin

- Salt and pepper to taste

- Fresh cilantro for garnish (optional)

- Cooked brown rice for serving

Directions:

1. In a large skillet, sauté chopped onion and minced garlic in a bit of olive oil until onion is translucent, about 3-4 minutes.

2. Add mixed vegetables to the skillet and sauté for another 5 minutes.

3. Stir in chickpeas, diced tomatoes, coconut milk, curry powder, cumin, salt, and pepper.

4. Simmer for 15-20 minutes, or until vegetables are tender and the sauce has thickened.

5. Serve hot over cooked brown rice.

6. Garnish with fresh cilantro if desired.

Nutritional Value (per serving):

- Calories: 380

- Protein: 11g

- Carbohydrates: 42g

- Fiber: 12g

- Fat: 21g

Recipe 46: Roasted Beet and Quinoa Salad with Orange Vinaigrette

Prep Time: 30 minutes

Serves: 4

Ingredients:

- 2 cups cooked quinoa, cooled

- 4 medium beets, roasted and diced

- 1/2 cup chopped walnuts, toasted

- 1/4 cup fresh parsley, chopped

- Juice and zest of 1 orange

- 2 tablespoons olive oil

- 1 tablespoon honey

- Salt and pepper to taste

Directions:

1. In a large bowl, combine cooked quinoa, roasted and diced beets, toasted chopped walnuts, and chopped fresh parsley.

2. In a small bowl, whisk together orange juice, orange zest, olive oil, honey, salt, and pepper.

3. Drizzle the orange vinaigrette over the salad and toss gently to combine.

4. Serve chilled.

Nutritional Value (per serving):

- Calories: 320

- Protein: 8g

- Carbohydrates: 37g

- Fiber: 6g

- Fat: 18g

Recipe 47: Mediterranean Stuffed Bell Peppers

Prep Time: 30 minutes

Serves: 4

Ingredients:

- 4 bell peppers, any color

- 1 cup cooked quinoa

- 1/2 cup canned chickpeas, drained and rinsed

- 1/2 cup diced cucumber

- 1/2 cup cherry tomatoes, halved

- 1/4 cup Kalamata olives, pitted and sliced

- 1/4 cup crumbled feta cheese

- 2 tablespoons extra-virgin olive oil

- Juice of 1 lemon

- 1 teaspoon dried oregano

- Salt and pepper to taste

Directions:

1. Preheat your oven to 375°F (190°C).

2. Cut the tops off the bell peppers and remove the seeds and membranes.

3. In a large bowl, combine cooked quinoa, chickpeas, diced cucumber, halved cherry tomatoes, sliced Kalamata olives, crumbled feta cheese, extra-virgin olive oil, lemon juice, dried oregano, salt, and pepper.

4. Stuff the bell peppers with the quinoa and vegetable mixture.

5. Place the stuffed peppers in a baking dish and cover with aluminum foil.

6. Bake for 25-30 minutes, or until the peppers are tender.

7. Serve hot.

Nutritional Value (per serving):

- Calories: 300

- Protein: 10g

- Carbohydrates: 39g

- Fiber: 8g

- Fat: 13g

Recipe 48: Turmeric and Ginger Lentil Soup

Prep Time: 30 minutes

Serves: 6

Ingredients:

- 2 cups green or brown lentils, rinsed and drained

- 1 onion, chopped

- 2 carrots, chopped

- 2 celery stalks, chopped

- 2 cloves garlic, minced

- 1 tablespoon fresh ginger, grated

- 1 tablespoon ground turmeric

- 8 cups vegetable broth

- Salt and pepper to taste

- Fresh cilantro for garnish (optional)

Directions:

1. In a large pot, sauté chopped onion, chopped carrots, chopped celery, minced garlic, and grated ginger in a bit of olive oil until vegetables begin to soften, about 5 minutes.

2. Add rinsed lentils, ground turmeric, vegetable broth, salt, and pepper to the pot.

3. Bring to a boil, then reduce heat and simmer for 20-25 minutes, or until lentils are tender.

4. Serve hot, garnished with fresh cilantro if desired.

Nutritional Value (per serving):

- Calories: 280

- Protein: 16g

- Carbohydrates: 49g

- Fiber: 16g

- Fat: 2g

Recipe 49: Lemon Rosemary Roasted Vegetables

Prep Time: 20 minutes

Serves: 4

Ingredients:

- 4 cups mixed vegetables (carrots, potatoes, Brussels sprouts)

- 2 tablespoons olive oil

- Juice and zest of 1 lemon

- 2 tablespoons fresh rosemary, chopped

- Salt and pepper to taste

Directions:

1. Preheat your oven to 425°F (220°C).

2. In a large bowl, toss mixed vegetables with olive oil, lemon juice, lemon zest, chopped fresh rosemary, salt, and pepper.

3. Spread the vegetables in a single layer on a baking sheet.

4. Roast for 20-25 minutes, or until the vegetables are tender and slightly crispy.

5. Serve hot.

Nutritional Value (per serving):

- Calories: 150

- Protein: 3g

- Carbohydrates: 19g

- Fiber: 5g

- Fat: 7g

Recipe 50: Avocado and Cucumber Soup

Prep Time: 15 minutes

Serves: 4

Ingredients:

- 2 avocados, peeled and pitted

- 2 cucumbers, peeled and chopped

- 1 cup Greek yogurt (unsweetened)

- 2 cups vegetable broth

- Juice of 2 limes

- 2 cloves garlic, minced

- Salt and pepper to taste

- Fresh cilantro for garnish (optional)

Directions:

1. In a blender, combine peeled and pitted avocados, chopped cucumbers, Greek yogurt, vegetable broth, lime juice, minced garlic, salt, and pepper.

2. Blend until smooth and creamy.

3. Serve chilled, garnished with fresh cilantro if desired.

Nutritional Value (per serving):

- Calories: 200

- Protein: 7g

- Carbohydrates: 17g

- Fiber: 9g

- Fat: 13g

Recipe 51: Mediterranean Quinoa Bowl

Prep Time: 20 minutes

Serves: 4

Ingredients:

- 2 cups cooked quinoa, cooled

- 1 cup cherry tomatoes, halved

- 1 cucumber, diced

- 1/2 cup Kalamata olives, pitted and sliced

- 1/4 cup red onion, finely chopped

- 1/4 cup crumbled feta cheese

- 2 tablespoons extra-virgin olive oil

- Juice of 1 lemon

- 1 teaspoon dried oregano

- Salt and pepper to taste

- Fresh parsley for garnish (optional)

Directions:

1. In a large bowl, combine cooked quinoa, halved cherry tomatoes, diced cucumber, sliced Kalamata olives, finely chopped red onion, and crumbled feta cheese.

2. In a small bowl, whisk together extra-virgin olive oil, lemon juice, dried oregano, salt, and pepper.

3. Drizzle the dressing over the quinoa bowl and toss gently to combine.

4. Serve chilled, garnished with fresh parsley if desired.

Nutritional Value (per serving):

- Calories: 300

- Protein: 7g

- Carbohydrates: 34g

- Fiber: 5g

- Fat: 16g

Recipe 52: Ginger and Turmeric Carrot Soup

Prep Time: 25 minutes

Serves: 6

Ingredients:

- 2 pounds carrots, peeled and chopped

- 1 onion, chopped

- 2 cloves garlic, minced

- 2 tablespoons fresh ginger, grated

- 1 tablespoon ground turmeric

- 6 cups vegetable broth

- 1 can (14 oz) coconut milk (unsweetened)

- 2 tablespoons olive oil

- Salt and pepper to taste

- Fresh cilantro for garnish (optional)

Directions:

1. In a large pot, sauté chopped onion, chopped carrots, minced garlic, and grated ginger in olive oil until vegetables begin to soften, about 5 minutes.

2. Add ground turmeric, vegetable broth, salt, and pepper to the pot.

3. Bring to a boil, then reduce heat and simmer for 20-25 minutes, or until carrots are tender.

4. Use an immersion blender to puree the soup until smooth. Alternatively, blend in batches in a regular blender.

5. Return the soup to the pot, add coconut milk, and heat gently.

6. Serve hot, garnished with fresh cilantro if desired.

Nutritional Value (per serving):

- Calories: 200

- Protein: 3g

- Carbohydrates: 17g

- Fiber: 4g

- Fat: 14g

Recipe 53: Spinach and Mushroom Stuffed Chicken Breast

Prep Time: 30 minutes

Serves: 4

Ingredients:

- 4 boneless, skinless chicken breasts

- 2 cups fresh spinach leaves

- 1 cup mushrooms, sliced

- 2 cloves garlic, minced

- 1/4 cup low-fat mozzarella cheese, shredded

- 1 tablespoon olive oil

- Salt and pepper to taste

Directions:

1. Preheat your oven to 375°F (190°C).

2. In a skillet, heat olive oil over medium heat. Add sliced mushrooms and minced garlic, sauté for 5-7 minutes until mushrooms are tender and any liquid has evaporated. Remove from heat.

3. Butterfly each chicken breast by making a horizontal cut, leaving one edge intact.

4. Open up the chicken breasts and place them between two sheets of plastic wrap. Pound them to an even thickness, about 1/2 inch.

5. Lay fresh spinach leaves on each chicken breast, followed by the sautéed mushrooms and shredded mozzarella cheese.

6. Fold the chicken breasts over to enclose the filling, securing with toothpicks if needed.

7. Season the stuffed chicken breasts with salt and pepper.

8. Place the chicken breasts in a baking dish and bake for 25-30 minutes, or until the chicken is cooked through and the cheese is melted and bubbly.

9. Serve hot.

Nutritional Value (per serving):

- Calories: 250

- Protein: 36g

- Carbohydrates: 4g

- Fiber: 1g

- Fat:

Recipe 54: Roasted Asparagus with Lemon and Almonds

Prep Time: 20 minutes

Serves: 4

Ingredients:

- 1 pound asparagus spears, trimmed

- 2 tablespoons olive oil

- Juice and zest of 1 lemon

- 1/4 cup sliced almonds, toasted

- Salt and pepper to taste

Directions:

1. Preheat your oven to 425°F (220°C).

2. Toss trimmed asparagus spears with olive oil, lemon juice, lemon zest, salt, and pepper.

3. Spread the asparagus on a baking sheet.

4. Roast for 10-15 minutes, or until tender and slightly crispy.

5. Sprinkle with toasted sliced almonds before serving.

Nutritional Value (per serving):

- Calories: 90

- Protein: 3g

- Carbohydrates: 5g

- Fiber: 3g

- Fat: 7g

Recipe 55: Herbed Quinoa and Chickpea Salad

Prep Time: 25 minutes

Serves: 4

Ingredients:

- 2 cups cooked quinoa, cooled

- 1 can (15 oz) chickpeas, drained and rinsed

- 1/2 cup chopped fresh herbs (such as parsley, mint, and cilantro)

- 1/4 cup red onion, finely chopped

- 2 tablespoons extra-virgin olive oil

- Juice of 1 lemon

- Salt and pepper to taste

Directions:

1. In a large bowl, combine cooked quinoa, chickpeas, chopped fresh herbs, finely chopped red onion, extra-virgin olive oil, lemon juice, salt, and pepper.

2. Toss to combine.

3. Serve chilled.

Nutritional Value (per serving):

- Calories: 280

- Protein: 9g

- Carbohydrates: 41g

- Fiber: 9g

- Fat: 10g

Recipe 56: Grilled Eggplant and Zucchini with Pesto

Prep Time: 30 minutes

Serves: 4

Ingredients:

- 1 eggplant, sliced

- 2 zucchinis, sliced

- 1/4 cup pesto sauce (store-bought or homemade)

- 2 tablespoons olive oil

- Salt and pepper to taste

- Fresh basil leaves for garnish (optional)

Directions:

1. Preheat your grill to medium-high heat.

2. In a bowl, toss eggplant and zucchini slices with olive oil, salt, and pepper.

3. Grill the slices for about 2-3 minutes per side until they have grill marks and are tender.

4. Remove from the grill and drizzle with pesto sauce.

5. Garnish with fresh basil leaves if desired.

6. Serve hot.

Nutritional Value (per serving):

- Calories: 190

- Protein: 3g

- Carbohydrates: 10g

- Fiber: 4g

- Fat: 16g

Recipe 57: Cilantro Lime Rice

Prep Time: 15 minutes

Serves: 4

Ingredients:

- 2 cups cooked brown rice, cooled

- 1/2 cup fresh cilantro, chopped

- Juice and zest of 2 limes

- 1 tablespoon olive oil

- Salt to taste

Directions:

1. In a bowl, combine cooked brown rice, chopped fresh cilantro, lime juice, lime zest, olive oil, and salt.

2. Toss to combine.

3. Serve chilled.

Nutritional Value (per serving):

- Calories: 180

- Protein: 3g

- Carbohydrates: 34g

- Fiber: 2g

- Fat: 4g

Recipe 58: Honey Glazed Salmon

Prep Time: 20 minutes

Serves: 4

Ingredients:

- 4 salmon fillets

- 2 tablespoons honey

- 1 tablespoon Dijon mustard

- 1 tablespoon low-sodium soy sauce

- 1 clove garlic, minced

- Salt and pepper to taste

- Lemon wedges for garnish (optional)

Directions:

1. In a bowl, whisk together honey, Dijon mustard, low-sodium soy sauce, minced garlic, salt, and pepper.

2. Brush the honey glaze over each salmon fillet.

3. Heat a skillet over medium-high heat and add a bit of olive oil.

4. Place the salmon fillets in the skillet, skin side down, and cook for 4-5 minutes per side, or until the salmon is cooked through and the glaze is caramelized.

5. Garnish with lemon wedges if desired.

6. Serve hot.

Nutritional Value (per serving):

- Calories: 260

- Protein: 24g

- Carbohydrates: 8g

- Fiber: 0g

- Fat: 15g

Recipe 59: Broccoli and Almond Salad *Prep*

Time: 15 minutes

Serves: 4

Ingredients:

- 4 cups broccoli florets, blanched and cooled

- 1/4 cup sliced almonds, toasted

- 1/4 cup dried cranberries

- 2 tablespoons Greek yogurt (unsweetened)

- 1 tablespoon mayonnaise (preferably low-fat)

- 1 tablespoon white wine vinegar

- Salt and pepper to taste

Directions:

1. In a large bowl, combine blanched and cooled broccoli florets, toasted sliced almonds, and dried cranberries.

2. In a small bowl, whisk together Greek yogurt, mayonnaise, white wine vinegar, salt, and pepper.

3. Drizzle the dressing over the salad and toss gently to combine.

4. Serve chilled.

Nutritional Value (per serving):

- Calories: 140

- Protein: 5g

- Carbohydrates: 17g

- Fiber: 4g

- Fat: 7g

Recipe 60: Grilled Portobello Mushrooms with Balsamic Glaze

Prep Time: 20 minutes

Serves: 4

Ingredients:

- 4 large portobello mushrooms

- 1/4 cup balsamic vinegar

- 2 tablespoons olive oil

- 2 cloves garlic, minced

- Salt and pepper to taste

- Fresh basil leaves for garnish (optional)

Directions:

1. Clean the portobello mushrooms and remove the stems.

2. In a bowl, whisk together balsamic vinegar, olive oil, minced garlic, salt, and pepper.

3. Brush the balsamic mixture over both sides of each mushroom.

4. Preheat your grill to medium-high heat.

5. Grill the mushrooms for about 4-5 minutes per side, or until they are tender and grill marks appear.

6. Remove from the grill and drizzle with any remaining balsamic glaze.

7. Garnish with fresh basil leaves if desired.

8. Serve hot.

Nutritional Value (per serving):

- Calories: 80

- Protein: 4g

- Carbohydrates: 8g

- Fiber: 2g

- Fat: 5g

CONCLUSION

As we come to the end of the "Anti-Cancer Diet Cookbook," we hope that this culinary journey has provided you with not only a collection of flavorful recipes but also valuable insights into the powerful role that food can play in our overall health and well-being.

Remember that the choices you make in your kitchen have the potential to shape your health and your future. By embracing a diet rich in cancer-fighting ingredients, you are taking proactive steps to reduce your risk of cancer and support your body in its fight against this formidable adversary.

While this cookbook offers a diverse range of recipes, it is just the beginning of your exploration into the world of wholesome and nutritious eating. We encourage you to continue learning about the incredible benefits of whole foods, experimenting with new ingredients, and making informed choices about what you put on your plate.

We also want to remind you that a healthy diet is just one aspect of a holistic approach to cancer prevention and well-being. Regular exercise, stress management, and a supportive network of friends and family all contribute to a healthier and happier life.

Lastly, we would like to express our gratitude for allowing us to be a part of your journey towards better health. Your commitment to taking charge of your diet is a powerful step towards a brighter and more vibrant future. We hope that the recipes in this cookbook have brought you joy, nourishment, and a deeper connection to the foods you consume.

As you continue on your path to a cancer-fighting lifestyle, remember that small changes can lead to significant results. Every meal is an opportunity to nourish your body and embrace a healthier you. We wish you continued success, vitality, and happiness on your journey, and we thank you for choosing the "Anti-Cancer Diet Cookbook" as your guide.

Here's to a future filled with good health, delicious meals, and the knowledge that you are taking charge of your well-being, one bite at a time. Cheers to a brighter and healthier you!

www.ingramcontent.com/pod-product-compliance
Lightning Source LLC
Chambersburg PA
CBHW050733260726
48661CB00001B/217